19494649R00063

Printed in Great Britain
by Amazon